ANTI AGING COOKBOOK FOR SENIORS

Quick and easy anti inflammatory recipes to promote longevity and healthy skin

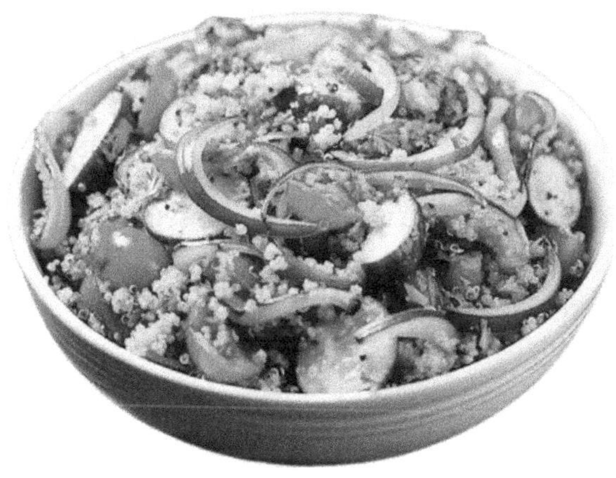

Dr. Malvin Harison

TABLE OF CONTENT

Introduction

Welcome to "Timeless Tastes: An Anti-Aging Cookbook for Seniors." Aging gracefully is not just a matter of passing years but a celebration of nourishing our bodies with the vitality they deserve. In this culinary journey, we invite you to savor the flavors of longevity, where every recipe is a testament to the art of aging well. Designed specifically for seniors, this cookbook is more than a collection of delicious dishes; it's a guide to embracing a lifestyle that enriches not just your palate, but your well-being. Let's embark on a gastronomic adventure that not only defies the hands of time but also celebrates the joy of savoring each moment. Get ready to relish the wisdom of age with every delightful bite!

Understanding Anti Aging Cookbook for Seniors

"Understanding Anti-Aging Cookbook for Seniors" delves into the science and art of nourishing the body to promote health, vitality, and graceful aging. This cookbook is more than just a compilation of recipes; it's a comprehensive guide that empowers seniors to make informed choices about their diet, embracing ingredients and culinary techniques that support well-being.

In this book, you'll discover:

1. Nutrient-Rich Recipes: Explore a diverse range of recipes carefully crafted to include ingredients rich in antioxidants, vitamins, and minerals known for their anti-aging properties. From vibrant salads to hearty stews, each dish is a flavorful journey towards a healthier you.

2. Understanding Aging: Gain insights into the aging process and how certain foods can positively impact longevity. Explore the science behind age-defying nutrients and how they contribute to maintaining cognitive function, supporting bone health, and enhancing overall vitality.

3. Practical Tips and Tricks: Beyond recipes, find practical tips and tricks for meal planning, grocery shopping, and creating a kitchen environment that fosters healthy eating habits. Learn how to make informed choices when it comes to portion sizes, cooking methods, and ingredient substitutions.

4. Culinary Adventures: Embark on a culinary adventure with inventive and delicious recipes that prove eating for anti-aging doesn't mean sacrificing flavor.

Discover new ingredients, cooking techniques, and flavor combinations that make every meal an enjoyable experience.

5. Lifestyle Integration: Recognize the importance of a holistic approach to anti-aging, including exercise, hydration, and stress management. This cookbook is a companion on your journey to a balanced and fulfilling lifestyle that promotes longevity.

The significance of adopting the right diet

The importance of anti-aging cookbooks among seniors cannot be overstated. Proper nutrition plays a pivotal role in promoting overall health, preventing age-related diseases, and enhancing the quality of life.

Here are key points highlighting the importance of a well-balanced diet for seniors:

1. Nutrient Absorption and Energy Levels: The right diet ensures seniors receive essential nutrients, vitamins, and minerals crucial for the body's proper functioning. Adequate nutrition helps maintain energy levels, preventing fatigue and promoting an active lifestyle.

2. Cognitive Function and Brain Health: Certain nutrients, such as omega-3 fatty acids and antioxidants found in fruits and vegetables, support cognitive function and may reduce the risk of cognitive decline in seniors. A well-balanced diet contributes to maintaining brain health and can positively impact memory and concentration.

3. Bone Health and Muscle Maintenance: Calcium and vitamin D, commonly found in dairy products and fortified foods, are vital for bone health, reducing the risk of osteoporosis and fractures. Protein intake is crucial for preserving muscle mass and strength, especially in aging individuals.

4. Immune System Support: Adequate nutrition supports a robust immune system, helping seniors fend off infections and illnesses. Nutrient-rich foods contribute to a well-functioning immune response, essential for overall health.

5. Digestive Health and Nutrient Absorption: A diet rich in fiber aids in digestion, preventing constipation and promoting a healthy gut microbiome. Proper nutrient absorption is facilitated by a well-functioning digestive system, ensuring seniors get the most benefit from their food.

Food to eat

A well-balanced and nutrient-dense diet is essential for anti-aging among seniors. Including a variety of foods rich in antioxidants, vitamins, minerals, and other essential nutrients can support overall health and well-being. Here are some recommendations for foods to eat for anti-aging seniors:

Foods to Eat

1. Colorful Fruits and Vegetables: Berries, leafy greens, carrots, and other colorful fruits and vegetables are rich in antioxidants that help combat oxidative stress and inflammation.

2. Fatty Fish: Salmon, mackerel, and sardines are high in omega-3 fatty acids, which support brain health and reduce the risk of chronic diseases.

3. Nuts and Seeds: Almonds, walnuts, chia seeds, and flax seeds provide healthy fats, fiber, and essential nutrients that contribute to heart health and overall well-being.

4. Whole Grains: Quinoa, brown rice, oats, and whole wheat provide fiber, vitamins, and minerals, promoting digestive health and sustained energy levels.

5. Lean Proteins: Skinless poultry, fish, tofu, beans, and legumes are excellent sources of protein, essential for muscle maintenance and overall body function.

6. Dairy or Dairy Alternatives: Low-fat or non-fat dairy, or fortified plant-based alternatives, provide calcium and vitamin D for bone health.

7. Healthy Fats: Avocado, olive oil, and nuts contain monounsaturated fats that support heart health and provide a source of energy.

8.   Probiotics: Yogurt, kefir, sauerkraut, and other fermented foods promote a healthy gut microbiome, supporting digestion and immune function.

9. Hydrating Beverages: Water, herbal teas, and infused water help maintain hydration, contributing to skin health and overall bodily functions.

10. Herbs and Spices: Turmeric, ginger, garlic, and other herbs and spices have anti-inflammatory properties and can add flavor without excessive salt or sugar.

Foods to Avoid

1. Processed Foods: Minimize the intake of processed and packaged foods, which often contain unhealthy trans fats, excessive sodium, and added sugars.

2. Sugary Snacks and Beverages: Limit the consumption of sugary snacks, desserts, and sweetened beverages, as excessive sugar intake may contribute to inflammation and other health issues.

3. Highly Processed Meats: Reduce the consumption of processed meats like sausages and bacon, which may contain preservatives and unhealthy additives.

4. Excessive Red and Processed Meats: While lean meats are beneficial, excessive consumption of red and processed meats has been linked to certain health risks. Opt for moderation.

5. Trans Fats: Avoid foods high in trans fats, often found in some margarines, fried foods, and commercially baked goods.

6. Excessive Alcohol: Limit alcohol consumption, as excessive drinking can contribute to dehydration and other health issues.

7. High-Sodium Foods: Reduce intake of high-sodium foods, as excess sodium can contribute to high blood pressure and other cardiovascular issues.

8. Empty-Calorie Foods: Minimize the consumption of foods with empty calories, lacking essential nutrients.

Chapter 1: Delicious Breakfast Recipes

Here are 10 delicious and nutrient-rich breakfast recipes that are easy to prepare and promote anti-aging management:

1. Green Smoothie Bowl

Ingredients:
- 1 cup spinach
- 1 frozen banana
- 1/2 avocado
- 1/2 cup almond milk
- 1 tablespoon chia seeds
- Toppings: sliced fruits, nuts, and seeds

Preparation:
1. Blend spinach, banana, avocado, almond milk, and chia seeds until smooth.
2. Pour the mixture into a bowl and add your favorite toppings.
3. Serve immediately.

Servings: 1

Nutritional Value (approx.):
- Calories: 350
- Protein: 8g
- Fiber: 12g
- Healthy fats: 18g
- Vitamins and minerals: High in Vitamin C, Vitamin E, Vitamin K, and potassium
Cooking time: 5 minutes

2. Overnight Chia Pudding

Ingredients:
- 3 tablespoons chia seeds
- 1 cup almond milk
- 1 tablespoon honey or maple syrup
- 1/2 teaspoon vanilla extract
- Fresh berries for topping

Preparation:

1. In a jar, combine chia seeds, almond milk, honey or maple syrup, and vanilla extract.

2. Stir well to combine, ensuring there are no clumps.

3. Refrigerate overnight or for at least 4 hours.

4. Before serving, give it a good stir and top with fresh berries.

Servings: 2

Nutritional Value (approx.):

- Calories: 180

- Protein: 6g

- Fiber: 10g

- Healthy fats: 8g

- Vitamins and minerals: High in Omega-3 fatty acids, calcium, and antioxidants

Cooking time: 5 minutes (plus refrigeration time)

3. Quinoa Breakfast Bowl

Ingredients:

- 1/2 cup cookcd quinoa

- 1/4 cup Greek yogurt

- 1 tablespoon almond butter

- 1 tablespoon honey or maple syrup

- Fresh fruits and nuts for topping

Preparation:

1. In a bowl, combine cooked quinoa, Greek yogurt, almond butter, and honey or maple syrup.

2. Mix well till all ingredients are well combined.

3. Top with fresh fruits and nuts of your choice.

Servings: 1

Nutritional Value (approx.):

- Calories: 400
- Protein: 15g
- Fiber: 8g
- Healthy fats: 10g
- Vitamins and minerals: High in iron, magnesium, and antioxidants

Cooking time: 10 minutes (assuming quinoa is pre-cooked)

4. Avocado Toast

Ingredients:

- 2 slices of whole-grain bread
- 1 ripe avocado
- 1 tablespoon lemon juice
- Salt and pepper to taste

Preparation:

1. Toast the bread slices until golden brown.

2. In a bowl, mash the avocado with lemon juice, salt, and pepper.

3. Spread the avocado mixture evenly on the toast.

Servings: 2

Nutritional Value (approx.):

- Calories (per serving): 200
- Protein: 6g
- Fiber: 8g
- Healthy fats: 10g
- Vitamins and minerals: High in Vitamin E, Vitamin K, and potassium

Cooking time: 10 minutes

5. Berry Oatmeal

Ingredients:

- 1/2 cup rolled oats
- 1 cup almond milk
- 1/2 cup mixed berries (fresh or frozen)
- 1 tablespoon honey or maple syrup
- 1 tablespoon almond butter or chopped nuts

Preparation:

1. In a saucepan, combine rolled oats and almond milk.

2. Cook over medium heat, stirring occasionally, until the oats are cooked and the mixture thickens.

3. Remove from heat and stir in mixed berries and honey or maple syrup.

4. Top with almond butter or chopped nuts.

Servings: 1

Nutritional Value (approx.):

- Calories: 300
- Protein: 8g
- Fiber: 7g
- Healthy fats: 10g
- Vitamins and minerals: High in antioxidants, Vitamin C, and Vitamin E

Cooking time: 10 minutes

6. Spinach and Mushroom Omelet

Ingredients:

- 2 eggs
- 1 cup spinach, chopped
- 1/2 cup mushrooms, sliced
- 1 tablespoon olive oil
- Salt and pepper to taste

Preparation:

1. In a bowl, beat the eggs with salt and pepper.

2. Heat olive oil in a non-stick pan over medium heat.

3. Add mushrooms and sauté until they release their moisture.

4. Add chopped spinach and cook until wilted.

5.5. Push the vegetables to one side of the pan and pour the beaten eggs into the other side.

6. Cook the eggs until they are set and lightly browned on the bottom.

7. Fold the omelet in half and cook for another minute.

8. Transfer to a plate and serve.

Servings: 1

Nutritional Value (approx.):

- Calories: 250
- Protein: 15g
- Fiber: 3g
- Healthy fats: 12g
- Vitamins and minerals: High in Vitamin A, Vitamin K, and iron

Cooking time: 10 minutes

7. Greek Yogurt Parfait

Ingredients:
- 1 cup Greek yogurt
- 1/4 cup granola
- 1/4 cup mixed berries
- 1 tablespoon honey or maple syrup

Preparation:
1. In a glass or bowl, layer Greek yogurt, granola, and mixed berries.
2. Drizzle with honey or maple syrup.

Servings: 1

Nutritional Value (approx.):
- Calories: 300
- Protein: 20g
- Fiber: 4g
- Healthy fats: 6g
- Vitamins and minerals: High in calcium, Vitamin C, and antioxidants

Preparation time: 5 minutes

8. Sweet Potato Pancakes

Ingredients:
- 1 cup cooked and mashed sweet potato
- 2 eggs
- 1/4 cup almond flour
- 1/2 teaspoon baking powder
- 1/2 teaspoon cinnamon
- Maple syrup for serving

Preparation:
1. In a bowl, combine mashed sweet potato, eggs, almond flour, baking powder, and cinnamon.
2. Combine very well till all ingredients are well mixed.
3. Heat a pan and lightly grease it.
4. Spread the batter onto the pot to make pancakes.
5. Cook until bubbles form on the surface, then flip and cook the other side.
6. Mizzle of maple syrup.

Servings: 2-3
Nutritional Value (approx.):
- Calories (per serving): 200
- Protein: 8g

- Fiber: 4g
- Healthy fats: 8g
- Vitamins and minerals: Vitamin A, Vitamin C, and potassium
Cooking time: 20 minutes

9. Salmon and Avocado Toast

Ingredients:
- 2 slices of whole-grain bread
- 2 ounces smoked salmon
- 1/2 avocado, sliced
- 1 tablespoon lemon juice
- Salt and pepper to taste

Preparation:
1. Toast the bread slices until golden brown.
2. In a small bowl, mash the avocado with lemon juice, salt, and pepper.
3. Spread the mashed avocado evenly on the toast.
4. Top with smoked salmon slices.

Servings: 2

Nutritional Value (approx.):
- Calories (per serving): 250
- Protein: 15g

- Fiber: 8g
- Healthy fats: 12g
- Vitamins and minerals: High in Omega-3 fatty acids, Vitamin D, and Vitamin E
Cooking time: 10 minutes

10. Veggie Egg Muffins

Ingredients:
- 6 eggs
- 1/2 cup chopped vegetables (such as spinach, bell peppers, tomatoes)
- 1/4 cup shredded cheese
- Salt and pepper to taste

Preparation:
1. Heat the oven to 175°C and grease a muffin tin.
2. In a bowl, beat the eggs with salt and pepper.
3. Divide the chopped vegetables evenly among the muffin cups.
4. Pour the beaten eggs over the vegetables, filling each cup about 3/4 full.

5. Sprinkle shredded cheese on top of each muffin cup.

6. Bake for 15-20 minutes or until the eggs are set and lightly golden.

7. Remove from the oven and let them cool slightly before removing from the muffin tin.

Servings: 6

Nutritional Value (approx.):

- Calories (per serving): 100

- Protein: 8g

- Fiber: 1g

- Healthy fats: 6g

- Vitamins and minerals: High in Vitamin A, Vitamin C, and calcium

Cooking time: 25 minutes

Chapter 2: Satisfying Lunch Recipes

Here are 10 delicious, nutrient-rich, and easy-to-prepare lunch recipes that are beneficial for anti-aging management:

1. Quinoa Salad with Avocado and Berries

Ingredients:
- 1 cup cooked quinoa
- 1 ripe avocado, diced
- 1 cup of different berries (blueberries, strawberries, raspberries)
- 2 tablespoons chopped walnuts
- 2 tablespoons lemon juice
- 1 tablespoon extra-virgin olive oil
- Salt and pepper to taste

Preparation:
1. In a bowl, combine the cooked quinoa, diced avocado, mixed berries, and chopped walnuts.

2. In another small bowl, mix together lemon juice, olive oil, salt, and pepper.
3. Drizzle the dressing over the quinoa mixture and toss gently to combine.
4. Serve chilled.
Servings: 2
Nutritional Value per Serving:
- Calories: 350
- Protein: 9g
- Fiber: 10g
- Healthy fats: 17g
- Vitamin C: 30% of daily value
- Antioxidants from berries
Cooking Time: 15 minutes

2. Salmon and Broccoli Stir-Fry

Ingredients:
- 2 salmon filets
- 2 cups broccoli florets
- 1 red bell pepper, sliced
- 2 cloves garlic, minced
- 1 tablespoon low-sodium soy sauce
- 1 tablespoon sesame oil
- 1 teaspoon grated ginger
- Sesame seeds for garnish

Preparation:

1. Heat sesame oil in a large pan.

2. Add garlic and ginger and sauté for 1-2 minutes.

3. Add salmon filets and cook for 3-4 minutes on each side until cooked through.

4. Extract the salmon from the skillet and put aside.

5. In the same skillet, add broccoli florets and red bell pepper. Stir-fry for 4-5 minutes until tender-crisp.

6. Add soy sauce and cooked salmon back to the skillet and toss to combine.

7. Sprinkle with sesame seeds and serve.

Servings: 2

Nutritional Value per Serving:

- Calories: 400
- Protein: 30g
- Omega-3 fatty acids from salmon
- Fiber: 7g
- Vitamin C: 150% of daily value

Cooking Time: 20 minutes

3. Spinach and Mushroom Omelette

Ingredients:
- 3 large eggs
- 1 cup fresh spinach leaves
- ½ cup sliced mushrooms
- 2 tablespoons grated Parmesan cheese
- 1 tablespoon olive oil
- Salt and pepper to taste

Preparation:
1. Heat olive oil in a skillet.
2. Add mushrooms and sauté until tender.
3. Add spinach leaves and cook until wilted.
4. In a bowl, beat the eggs and season with salt and pepper.
5. Pour the beaten eggs into the skillet, covering the vegetables.
6. Cook for 2-3 minutes until the bottom is set.
7. Sprinkle Parmesan cheese over one half of the omelet and fold the other half over.
8. Cook for another minute until the cheese melts.

9. Slide the omelet onto a plate and serve.

Servings: 1

Nutritional Value per Serving:
- Calories: 300
- Protein: 20g
- Vitamin A: 90% of daily value
- Vitamin D: 15% of daily value
- Calcium: 20% of daily value

Cooking Time: 10 minutes

4. Lentil and Vegetable Soup:

Ingredients:
- 1 cup dried lentils, rinsed
- 1 carrot, diced
- 1 celery stalk, diced
- 1 onion, diced
- 2 cloves garlic, minced
- 4 cups low-sodium vegetable broth
- 1 teaspoon cumin
- 1 teaspoon turmeric
- 1 tablespoon olive oil
- Salt and pepper to taste

Preparation:

1. Heat olive oil in a big pot over small heat.

2. Add onions, carrots, celery, and garlic. Sauté for 5 minutes until vegetables soften.

3. Add lentils, vegetable broth, cumin, turmeric, salt, and pepper.

4. Bring the mixture to a boil, then reduce heat and simmer for 25-30 minutes until lentils are tender.

5. Adjust seasoning if needed.

6. Serve hot.

Servings: 4

Nutritional Value per Serving:

- Calories: 250
- Protein: 15g
- Fiber: 15g
- Folate: 50% of daily value
- Iron: 20% of daily value

Cooking Time: 40 minutes

5. Greek Salad

Ingredients

- 2 cups mixed salad greens
- 1 cucumber, sliced
- 1 cup cherry tomatoes, halved
- 1/4 red onion, thinly sliced
- 1/4 cup Kalamata olives
- 2 tablespoons crumbled feta cheese
- 1 tablespoon extra-virgin olive oil
- 1 tablespoon lemon juice
- 1 teaspoon dried oregano
- Salt and pepper to taste

Preparation:

1. In a large bowl, combine mixed salad greens, cucumber slices, cherry tomatoes, red onion slices, and Kalamata olives.

2. In a small bowl, whisk together olive oil, lemon juice, dried oregano, salt, and pepper to make the dressing.

3. Sprinkle the dressing all over the salad and toss to coat.

4. Sprinkle crumbled feta cheese on top.

5. Serve chilled.

Servings: 2

Nutritional Value per Serving:
- Calories: 200
- Protein: 5g
- Fiber: 4g
- Vitamin C: 40% of daily value
- Fats from olives and olive oil
Cooking Time: 10 minutes

6. Sweet Potato and Chickpea Buddha Bowl:

Ingredients:
- 1 large sweet potato, cubed
- 1 cup cooked chickpeas
- 2 cups baby spinach
- 1/4 cup diced red bell pepper
- 1/4 cup diced cucumber
- 2 tablespoons tahini
- 2 tablespoons lemon juice
- 1 tablespoon extra-virgin olive oil
- 1 teaspoon ground cumin
- Salt and pepper to taste
Preparation:
1. Preheat the oven to 400°F (200°C).
2. Toss sweet potato cubes with olive oil, cumin, salt, and pepper.

3. Spread the sweet potato cubes on a baking sheet and roast for 20-25 minutes until tender.

4. In a bowl, combine baby spinach, chickpeas, red bell pepper, and cucumber.

5. In a separate small bowl, whisk together tahini, lemon juice, olive oil, salt, and pepper to make the dressing.

6. Add the roasted sweet potatoes to the bowl of vegetables and drizzle with the dressing.

7. Toss gently to combine.

8. Serve at room temperature.

Servings: 2

Nutritional Value per Serving:

- Calories: 400
- Protein: 10g
- Fiber: 12g
- Vitamin A: 350% of daily value
- Vitamin K: 150% of daily value
- Iron: 15% of daily value

Cooking Time: 30 minutes

7. Quinoa Stuffed Bell Peppers:

Ingredients:
- 2 large bell peppers
- 1 cup cooked quinoa
- 1/2 cup black beans, rinsed and drained
- 1/4 cup corn kernels
- 1/4 cup diced tomatoes
- 1/4 cup shredded mozzarella cheese
- 1 teaspoon olive oil
- 1 teaspoon chili powder
- Salt and pepper to taste

Preparation:
1. Preheat the oven to 375°F (190°C).
2. Eliminate the bell peppers tops, the seeds and membranes.
3. In a bowl, combine cooked quinoa, black beans, corn kernels, diced tomatoes, olive oil, chili powder, salt, and pepper.
4. Stuff the bell peppers with the quinoa mixture and place them in a baking dish.
5. Bake for 25-30 minutes until the peppers are tender and the filling is heated through.

6. Sprinkle shredded mozzarella cheese on top and bake for an additional 5 minutes until the cheese is melted and golden.

7. Serve hot.

Servings: 2

Nutritional Value per Serving:

- Calories: 300
- Protein: 12g
- Fiber: 10g
- Vitamin C: 200% of daily value
- Antioxidants from bell peppers

Cooking Time: 45 minutes

8. Mediterranean Tuna Salad Wrap:

Ingredients:

- 1 can tuna in water, drained
- 1 tablespoon Greek yogurt
- 1 tablespoon lemon juice
- 1 tablespoon chopped fresh dill
- 1/4 cup diced cucumber
- 1/4 cup diced red onion
- 1/4 cup diced tomatoes
- 2 large lettuce leaves
- 2 whole-grain tortillas

Preparation:

1. In a bowl, combine tuna, Greek yogurt, lemon juice, chopped dill, diced cucumber, red onion, and tomatoes.

2. Mix well to combine.

3. Lay the lettuce leaves on the tortillas.

4. Spoon the tuna salad mixture onto the lettuce leaves.

5. Roll up the tortillas tightly to form wraps.

Servings: 2

Nutritional Value per Serving:

- Calories: 350
- Protein: 30g
- Fiber: 6g
- Vitamin C: 200% of daily value
- Antioxidants from colorful vegetables

Cooking Time: 20 minutes

9. Grilled Chicken and Vegetable Skewers:

Ingredients:

- 2 boneless, chicken breasts, cut into pieces
- 1 red bell pepper, cut into cubes

- 1 yellow bell pepper, cut into chunks
- 1 zucchini, sliced
- 1 red onion, cut into chunks
- 2 tablespoons olive oil
- 1 tablespoon balsamic vinegar
- 1 teaspoon dried Italian seasoning
- Salt and pepper to taste

Preparation:

1. Preheat the grill to medium-high heat.

2. In a bowl, combine olive oil, balsamic vinegar, dried Italian seasoning, salt, and pepper.

3. Thread the chicken, bell peppers, zucchini, and red onion onto skewers.

4. Drizzle the skewers with mixture of olive oil.

5. Grill the skewers for 10-12 minutes, turning occasionally until the chicken is cooked through and the vegetables are tender.

6. Serve hot.

Servings: 2

Nutritional Value per Serving:

- Calories: 350
- Protein: 30g

- Fiber: 6g
- Vitamin C: 200% of daily value
- Antioxidants from colorful vegetables
Cooking Time: 20 minutes

10. Berry Smoothie Bowl:

Ingredients
- 1 frozen banana
- 1 cup of different berries (blueberries, strawberries, raspberries)
- 1/2 cup almond milk
- 1 tablespoon chia seeds
- Toppings: sliced banana, mixed berries, granola, shredded coconut

Preparation
1. In a blender, combine the frozen banana, mixed berries, almond milk, and chia seeds.
2. Blend until smooth and creamy.
3. Pour the smoothie into a bowl.
4. Top with sliced banana, mixed berries, granola, and shredded coconut.
5. Serve immediately.

Servings: 1
Nutritional Value per Serving:

- Calories: 300
- Protein: 5g
- Fiber: 10g
- Vitamin C: 100% of daily value
- Antioxidants from berries
- Omega-3 fatty acids from chia seeds
Preparation Time: 5 minutes

Chapter 3: Nutritious Dinner Recipes

Here are 10 delicious, nutrient-rich, and easy-to-prepare dinner recipes that are anti-aging friendly, incorporating scientifically proven ingredients known for their anti-aging properties:

1. Turmeric-Ginger Baked Salmon

Ingredients:
- 4 salmon filets
- 1 tablespoon turmeric powder
- 1 tablespoon grated fresh ginger
- 2 cloves garlic, minced
- 1 tablespoon lemon juice
- Salt and pepper to taste
- Fresh cilantro for garnish

Preparation:
1. Preheat the oven to 375°F (190°C).

2. In a small bowl, mix turmeric powder, ginger, garlic, lemon juice, salt, and pepper.

3. Put the salmon filets on a baking tray lined with parchment paper.

4. Spread the turmeric-ginger mixture evenly over the salmon filets.

5. Bake for 12-15 minutes or until the salmon is cooked through.

6. Garnish with fresh cilantro before serving.

Servings: 4

Nutritional Value per Serving:

- Calories: 250
- Protein: 30g
- Fat: 12g
- Carbohydrates: 2g
- Fiber: 1g
- **Cooking Time**: 15 minutes

2. Quinoa-Stuffed Bell Peppers

Ingredients:

- 4 bell peppers (any color)
- 1 cup cooked quinoa

- 1 cup diced mixed vegetables (carrots, zucchini, mushrooms, etc.)
- 1/2 cup chopped onion
- 2 cloves garlic, minced
- 1 tablespoon olive oil
- 1 teaspoon dried oregano
- Salt and pepper to taste
- Grated Parmesan cheese (optional)

Preparation:

1. Preheat the oven to 375°F (190°C).

2. Remove the tops of the bell peppers and eliminate the seeds and membranes.

3. In a pan , heat olive oil over medium heat. Cook onions and garlic until translucent.

4. Add the mixed vegetables and cook until tender.

5. Stir in the cooked quinoa, dried oregano, salt, and pepper. Cook for another 2 minutes.

6. Stuff the bell peppers with the quinoa-vegetable mixture and place them in a baking dish.

7. Cover the dish with foil and bake for 25-30 minutes.

8. Remove the foil, sprinkle with grated Parmesan cheese (if desired), and bake for an additional 5 minutes until the cheese is melted and golden.

Servings: 4

Nutritional Value per Serving:
- Calories: 200
- Protein: 6g
- Fat: 5g
- Carbohydrates: 35g
- Fiber: 7g
- **Cooking Time**: 35 minutes

3. Garlic Herb Roasted Chicken with Vegetables

Ingredients:
- 4 boneless, chicken breasts
- 1 pound baby potatoes, halved
- 1 cup baby carrots
- 1 cup green beans, trimmed
- 2 cloves garlic, minced
- 3 tablespoons fresh spicy (rosemary, thyme, or parsley), cutted

- 2 tablespoons olive oil
- Salt and pepper to taste

Preparation:

1. Preheat the oven to 425°F (220°C).

2. In a large bowl, combine minced garlic, chopped herbs, olive oil, salt, and pepper.

3. Add chicken breasts, potatoes, carrots, and green beans to the bowl, and toss until well coated.

4. Transfer the chicken and vegetables to a baking dish, arranging them in a single layer.

5. Bake for 25-30 minutes or until the chicken is cooked through and the vegetables are tender.

6. Serve hot.

Servings: 4

Nutritional Value per Serving:

- Calories: 320
- Protein: 30g
- Fat: 10g
- Carbohydrates: 25g
- Fiber: 5g
- **Cooking Time**: 30 minutes

4. Spinach and Mushroom Quiche

Ingredients:
- 1 pre-made pie crust
- 4 cups fresh spinach, roughly chopped
- 1 cup sliced mushrooms
- 1 small onion, diced
- 4 eggs
- 1 cup milk
- 1 cup Gruyere or Swiss cheese(shredded)
- Salt and pepper to taste

Preparation:
1. Preheat the oven to 375°F (190°C).
2. Place the pie crust in a pie dish and set aside.
3. In a skillet, sauté onions and mushrooms until softened.
4. Add the chopped spinach and cook until wilted. Remove from heat.
5. In a mixing bowl, whisk together the eggs and milk. Season with salt and pepper.
6. Stir in the cooked vegetables and shredded cheese.

7. Put the mixture into the crust of the pie .

8. Bake for 35-40 minutes or until the quiche is set and golden brown.

9. Permit it to cool for some minutes before slicing and serving.

Servings: 6

Nutritional Value per Serving:

- Calories: 300
- Protein: 12g
- Fat: 18g
- Carbohydrates: 22g
- Fiber: 2g
- **Cooking Time**: 40 minutes

5. Kale and White Bean Soup

Ingredients:

- 1 tablespoon olive oil
- 1 onion, diced
- 2 cloves garlic, minced
- 4 cups vegetable broth
- 2 cups water
- 2 cups chopped kale
- 1 can (15 ounces) white beans, drained and rinsed

- 1 teaspoon dried thyme

- Salt and pepper to taste

- Grated Parmesan cheese for garnish (optional)

Preparation

1. In a big pot, heat olive oil. Add diced onions and minced garlic. Sauté until onions are translucent.

2. Add vegetable broth, water, chopped kale, white beans, dried thyme, salt, and pepper.

3. Bring the soup to a boil, then reduce heat and let it simmer for 15-20 minutes.

4. Adjust seasoning if needed.

5. Serve warm, add grated Parmesan cheese if desired.

Servings: 4

Nutritional Value per Serving:

- Calories: 180

- Protein: 8g

- Fat: 4g

- Carbohydrates: 29g

- Fiber: 8g

- **Cooking Time:** 30 minutes

6. Grilled Chicken with Roasted Vegetables

Ingredients:
- 4 boneless, skinless chicken breasts
- 2 cups broccoli florets
- 2 cups cauliflower florets
- 1 red bell pepper, sliced
- 1 yellow bell pepper, sliced
- 1 small red onion, sliced
- 2 tablespoons olive oil
- 2 cloves garlic, minced
- 1 teaspoon dried Italian seasoning
- Salt and pepper to taste

Preparation:
1. Preheat the grill to medium-high heat.
2. In a large bowl, combine broccoli florets, cauliflower florets, bell peppers, red onion, minced garlic, dried Italian seasoning, salt, pepper, and olive oil.
3. Grill the chicken breasts for about 6-8 minutes on each side or until cooked through.
4. Spread the seasoned vegetables on a baking sheet and roast in the oven at

400°F (200°C) for approximately 20-25 minutes or until tender.

5. Serve the grilled chicken with the roasted vegetables on the side.

Servings: 4

Nutritional Value per Serving:
- Calories: 280
- Protein: 35g
- Fat: 10g
- Carbohydrates: 15g
- Fiber: 5g
- **Cooking Time**: 35 minutes

7. Lentil and Vegetable Stir-Fry

Ingredients:
- 1 cup dried lentils
- 2 cups vegetable broth
- 1 tablespoon sesame oil
- 1 onion, thinly sliced
- 2 cloves garlic, minced
- 1 red bell pepper, thinly sliced
- 1 yellow bell pepper, thinly sliced
- 2 cups broccoli florets
- 1 cup snap peas
- 2 tablespoons low-sodium soy sauce

- 1 tablespoon rice vinegar
- 1 teaspoon honey
- 1 teaspoon grated fresh ginger
- Sesame seeds for garnish (optional)

Preparation:

1. Rinse the lentils and place them in a saucepan with vegetable broth. Place on fire to a boil, then deduce heat and simmer until lentils are soft. Drain any excess liquid and place aside.

2. In a large skillet or wok, heat sesame oil over medium heat. Add sliced onions and minced garlic, and sauté until fragrant and slightly softened.

3. Add the bell peppers, broccoli florets, and snap peas. Stir-fry for 5-6 minutes or until the vegetables are crisp-tender.

4. In a small bowl, whisk together soy sauce, rice vinegar, honey, and grated ginger.

5. Add cooked lentils and the sauce mixture to the skillet. Stir-fry for about 2-3 minutes until everything is well mixed.

6. Garnish with sesame seeds if desired and serve hot.

Servings: 4

Nutritional Value per Serving:

- Calories: 320
- Protein: 18g
- Fat: 4g
- Carbohydrates: 55g
- Fiber: 16g
- **Cooking Time:** 35 minutes

8. Berry and Spinach Salad with Citrus Vinaigrette

Ingredients:

- 4 cups fresh spinach leaves
- 1 cup mixed berries (strawberries, blueberries, raspberries)
- 1/4 cup sliced almonds
- 2 tablespoons crumbled feta cheese (optional)
- 2 tablespoons olive oil
- 1 tablespoon freshly squeezed orange juice
- 1 tablespoon freshly squeezed lemon juice

- 1 teaspoon honey
- Salt and pepper to taste

Preparation:

1. In a large salad bowl, combine fresh spinach leaves, mixed berries, sliced almonds, and crumbled feta cheese (if using).

2. In a separate small bowl, whisk together olive oil, orange juice, lemon juice, honey, salt, and pepper to make the citrus vinaigrette.

3. Drizzle the vinaigrette over the salad and toss gently to coat all the ingredients.

4. Serve immediately.

Servings: 4

Nutritional Value per Serving:

- Calories: 120
- Protein: 3g
- Fat: 8g
- Carbohydrates: 10g
- Fiber: 3g
- **Cooking Time**: 10 minutes

9. Chia Seed Pudding

Ingredients:
- 1/4 cup chia seeds
- 1 cup almond milk (unsweetened)
- 1 tablespoon honey or maple syrup
- 1/2 teaspoon vanilla extract
- Assorted fresh fruits for topping (berries, sliced banana, etc.)
- Nuts or seeds for topping (optional)

Preparation

1. In a bowl, combine chia seeds, almond milk, honey or maple syrup, and vanilla extract.

2. Mix thoroughly to make sure the chia seeds are evenly distributed.

3. Cover the bowl and keep it in the fridge overnight, allowing the chia seeds to absorb the liquid consistency.

4. Before serving, give the mixture a good stir to break up any clumps.

5. Divide the chia seed pudding into serving bowls and top with fresh fruits and nuts or seeds.

6. Enjoy chilled.

Servings: 2

Nutritional Value per Serving:

- Calories: 180
- Protein: 5g
- Fat: 9g
- Carbohydrates: 20g
- Fiber: 11g
- **Cooking Time**: 2 hours (chilling time)

10. Dark Chocolate Avocado Mousse

Ingredients:

- 2 ripe avocados
- 1/4 cup unsweetened cocoa powder
- 1/4 cup maple syrup or honey
- 1/4 cup almond milk (unsweetened)
- 1 teaspoon vanilla extract
- Fresh berries for garnish (optional)
- Shredded dark chocolate for garnish (optional)

Preparation:

1. Pill out the flesh of the avocados and place them in a blender.

2. Add cocoa powder, maple syrup or honey, almond milk, and vanilla extract to the blender.

3. Blend until smooth and creamy, scraping down the sides as needed.

4. Transfer the avocado mousse to serving glasses or bowls.

5. Chill in the refrigerator for at least 1 hour to firm up.

6. Garnish with fresh berries and shredded dark chocolate before serving.

Servings: 4

Nutritional Value per Serving:

- Calories: 200

- Protein: 3g

- Fat: 15g

- Carbohydrates: 20g

- Fiber: 8g

- **Cooking Time:** 1 hour (chilling time)

Chapter 4: Flavorful Snacks and Dessert Recipes

1. Berry Chia Pudding

Ingredients:

1 cup of different berries (blueberries, strawberries, raspberries)

2 tablespoons chia seeds

1 cup almond milk (unsweetened)

1 tablespoon honey or maple syrup (optional)

1/4 teaspoon vanilla extract

Preparation:

1. In a blender, blend the mixed berries until smooth.

2. In a bowl, combine the blended berries, chia seeds, almond milk, honey or maple syrup (if using), and vanilla extract. Stir well.

3. Cover the bowl and keep it in the fridge overnight.

4. Serve chilled.

Number of servings: 2
Nutritional value per serving:
- Calories: 120
- Protein: 4g
- Fat: 5g
- Carbohydrates: 16g
- Fiber: 9g
- Vitamin C: 50% of the daily value
- Antioxidants from berries
Cooking time: 5 minutes

2. Avocado Toast

Ingredients:
1 ripe avocado
2 slices whole grain bread
1/2 lemon
Salt and pepper to taste
Optional toppings: cherry tomatoes, sprouts, or sliced radishes
Preparation:
1. Toast the slices of bread.
2. Cut the avocado in into two, eliminate the pit, and put the flesh into a bowl.

3. Squeeze the juice of half a lemon over the avocado and mash it with a fork until creamy.

4. Season with salt and pepper to taste.

5. Spread the avocado mixture evenly on the toasted bread slices.

6. Top with optional toppings, if desired.

Number of servings: 2

Nutritional value per serving:

- Calories: 220

- Protein: 6g

- Fat: 12g

- Carbohydrates: 26g

- Fiber: 10g

- Vitamin E: 20% of the daily value

- Healthy fats from avocado

Cooking time: 10 minutes

3. Greek Yogurt Parfait

Ingredients

1 cup Greek yogurt (plain or flavored)

1/4 cup granola

1/4 cup mixed berries

1 tablespoon honey or maple syrup (optional)

Preparation

1. In a glass or bowl, layer the Greek yogurt, granola, and mixed berries.
2. Drizzle honey or maple syrup on top if desired.
3. Repeat the layers.
4. Serve immediately.

Number of servings: 1

Nutritional value per serving:

- Calories: 300
- Protein: 20g
- Fat: 6g
- Carbohydrates: 45g
- Fiber: 5g
- Calcium: 20% of the daily value
- Probiotics from Greek yogurt

Cooking time: 5 minutes

4. Roasted Chickpeas

Ingredients:

15 ounce chickpeas (1 can), washed and rinsed

1 tablespoon olive oil

1/2 teaspoon garlic powder

1/2 teaspoon paprika

1/4 teaspoon salt

1/4 teaspoon black pepper

Preparation:

1. Preheat the oven to 400°F (200°C).

2. In a bowl, toss the chickpeas with olive oil, garlic powder, paprika, salt, and black pepper until well coated.

3. Spread the chickpeas in a single layer on a baking sheet.

4. Roast in the oven for 20-25 minutes, shaking the baking sheet halfway through.

5. Remove from the oven and let them cool before serving.

Number of servings: 4

Nutritional value per serving:

- Calories: 130
- Protein: 6g
- Fat: 5g
- Carbohydrates: 16g
- Fiber: 5g
- Iron: 10% of the daily value
- Antioxidants from chickpeas

Cooking time: 25 minutes

5. Spinach and Feta Stuffed Mushrooms

Ingredients:

8 large button mushrooms

2 cups fresh spinach, chopped

1/4 cup crumbled feta cheese

1 clove garlic, minced

1 tablespoon olive oil

Salt and pepper to taste

Preparation:

1. Preheat the oven to 375°F (190°C).

2. Eliminate the stems from the mushrooms and place aside.

3. In a pan, heat olive oil. Add the mushroom stems, minced garlic, and chopped spinach. Cook until the spinach wilts.

4. Remove from heat and stir in the crumbled feta cheese.

5. Add salt and pepper to taste.

6. Stuff each mushroom cap with the spinach and feta mixture.

7. Place the stuffed mushroom on a baking sheet and bake for 15-20 minutes until the mushrooms are tender.

8. Serve hot.

Number of servings: 4

Nutritional value per serving:

- Calories: 80

- Protein: 4g

- Fat: 4g

- Carbohydrates: 7g

- Fiber: 2g

- Vitamin A: 60% of the daily value

- Antioxidants from spinach

Cooking time: 25 minutes

6. Quinoa Salad

Ingredients

1 cup cooked quinoa

1 cup of different vegetables (bell peppers, cucumber, cherry tomatoes)

3 tablespoons cutted fresh spicy (parsley, cilantro, or basil)

1 tablespoon lemon juice

1 tablespoon olive oil

Salt and pepper to taste

Preparation:

1. In a bowl, combine cooked quinoa, mixed vegetables, and chopped fresh herbs.

2. In a small bowl, whisk together lemon juice, olive oil, salt, and pepper.

3. Sprinkle the dressing over the quinoa and vegetables.

4. Toss well to combine.

5. Serve chilled or at room temperature.

Number of servings: 2

Nutritional value per serving:

- Calories: 250

- Protein: 8g

- Fat: 8g

- Carbohydrates: 35g

- Fiber: 6g

- Vitamin C: 80% of the daily value

- Antioxidants from vegetables

Cooking time: 20 minutes

7. Baked Sweet Potato Fries

Ingredients:

2 medium sweet potatoes

1 tablespoon olive oil

1/2 teaspoon paprika

1/2 teaspoon garlic powder

1/4 teaspoon salt

1/4 teaspoon black pepper

Preparation:

1. Preheat the oven to 425°F (220°C).

2. Peel the sweet potatoes and cut them into thin strips.

3. In a bowl, toss the sweet potato strips with olive oil, paprika, garlic powder, salt, and black pepper until well coated.

4. Spread the sweet potato strips in a single layer on a baking sheet.

5. Bake in the oven for 20-25 minutes, flipping halfway through, until the fries are crispy and golden brown.

6. Remove from the oven and let them cool slightly before serving.

Number of servings: 4

Nutritional value per serving:

- Calories: 100

- Protein: 2g
- Fat: 3g
- Carbohydrates: 18g
- Fiber: 3g
- Vitamin A: 200% of the daily value
- Beta-carotene from sweet potatoes
Cooking time: 25 minutes

8. Green Smoothie

Ingredients:

1 cup spinach or kale

1/2 medium banana

1/2 cup frozen mixed berries

1/2 cup almond milk (unsweetened)

1 tablespoon chia seeds

Preparation:

1. In a blender, combine spinach or kale, banana, frozen mixed berries, almond milk, and chia seeds.

2. Blend until smooth and creamy.

3. Add more almond milk if needed to reach the desired consistency.

4. Serve immediately.

Number of servings: 1

Nutritional value per serving:

- Calories: 180
- Protein: 5g
- Fat: 6g
- Carbohydrates: 28g
- Fiber: 9g
- Vitamin K: 200% of the daily value
- Antioxidants from greens and berries

Cooking time: 5 minutes

9. Dark Chocolate Energy Balls

Ingredients

1 cup Medjool dates, pitted

1/2 cup almonds

2 tablespoons unsweetened cocoa powder

1 tablespoon chia seeds

1 tablespoon honey or maple syrup

1/2 teaspoon vanilla extract

1/4 cup shredded coconut (optional)

Preparation

1. In a food processor, process dates and almonds until finely chopped.

2. Add cocoa powder, chia seeds, honey or maple syrup, and vanilla extract.

Process until the mixture comes together.

3. Turn the mixture into small balls utilizing your hands.

4. Optional: Roll the energy balls in shredded coconut to coat.

5. Keep in the fridge for at least 1 hour before serving.

Number of servings: 6

Nutritional value per serving (2 energy balls)

- Calories: 160
- Protein: 3g
- Fat: 7g
- Carbohydrates: 24g
- Fiber: 4g
- Iron: 10% of the daily value
- Antioxidants from dark chocolate

Cooking time: 15 minutes

10. Mango Yogurt Smoothie

Ingredients

1 ripe mango, peeled and pitted

1 cup Greek yogurt (plain or flavored)

1/2 cup almond milk (unsweetened)

1 tablespoon honey or maple syrup (optional)

1/2 teaspoon turmeric powder (optional)

Preparation

1. In a blender, combine the mango, Greek yogurt, almond milk, honey or maple syrup (if using), and turmeric powder (if using).

2. Blend until smooth and creamy.

3. Add more almond milk if needed to achieve the desired consistency.

4. Pour into glasses and serve chilled.

Number of servings: 2

Nutritional value per serving

- Calories: 180
- Protein: 10g
- Fat: 2g
- Carbohydrates: 34g
- Fiber: 3g
- Vitamin C: 100% of the daily value
- Probiotics from Greek yogurt
- Antioxidants from mango

Cooking time: 5 minutes

Chapter 5: Bonus 1

A 7- days Sample Meal Plan

Here's a sample 7-day meal plan for an anti-aging management cookbook for seniors:

Day 1

Breakfast: Vegetable omelet
Lunch: Grilled salmon with broccoli and quinoa.
Dinner: Roasted sweet potatoes fry's
Snack: Greek yogurt with mixed berries.

Day 2

Breakfast: Overnight Chia seeds pudding
Lunch: Quinoa and black bean salad
Dinner: Grilled tofu with stir-fried vegetables
Snack: Carrot sticks with hummus.

Day 3

Breakfast: Whole grain toast
Lunch: Lentil soup
Dinner: Baked cod.
Snack: Handful of walnuts.

Day 4

Breakfast: Spinach and mushroom frittata.
Lunch: Grilled chicken salad
Dinner: Zucchini noodles and marinara sauce.
Snack: Sliced apples with almond butter.

Day 5

Breakfast: Smoothie made with spinach, banana, almond milk, and a scoop of protein powder.
Lunch: Quinoa-stuffed bell peppers with a side of steamed asparagus.
Dinner: Baked salmon and brown rice.
Snack: Trail mix

Day 6

Breakfast: Whole grain pancakes
Lunch: Chickpea salad
Dinner: Grilled shrimp skewers
Snack: Celery sticks with almond butter.

Day 7

Breakfast: Veggie and egg scramble
Lunch: Quinoa and roasted vegetable bowl
Dinner: Baked chicken thigh
Snack: Sliced cucumbers with tzatziki sauce

Chapter 6: Bonus 2

20 Juicing and Smoothie Recipes for Anti Aging

Here are 10 juicing recipes and 10 smoothie recipes for anti-aging seniors:

1. Green Goddess

Ingredients: Spinach, cucumber, kale, green apple, lemon
Instructions: Blend all the ingredients together and serve.

2. Berry Blast

Ingredients: Blueberries, strawberries, raspberries, spinach, almond milk
Instructions: Juice the berries and spinach, then blend with almond milk.

3. Citrus Delight

Ingredients: Oranges, carrots, ginger
Instructions: Juice the oranges, carrots, and ginger together and enjoy.

4. Beet Booster

Ingredients: Beets, celery, apple, lemon
Instructions: Juice all the ingredients and drink immediately.

5. Mango Tango

Ingredients: Mango, pineapple, spinach, coconut water
Instructions: Juice the mango, pineapple, and spinach, then blend with coconut water.

6. Carrot Cleanser

Ingredients: Carrots, parsley, lemon
Instructions: Juice the carrots, parsley, and lemon together and serve.

7. Cucumber Cooler:

Ingredients: Cucumber, mint, lime
Instructions: Juice the cucumber, mint, and lime, then enjoy.

8. Tropical Paradise

Ingredients: Pineapple, kiwi, kale, coconut water
Instructions: Juice the pineapple, kiwi, and kale, then blend with coconut water.

9. Ginger Zinger

Ingredients: Apples, ginger, lemon
Instructions: Juice the apples, ginger, and lemon together and drink immediately.

10. Watermelon Refresher

Ingredients: Watermelon, mint, lime
Instructions: Juice the watermelon, mint, and lime, then serve.

11. Blueberry Bliss

Ingredients: Blueberries, Greek yogurt, almond milk, honey
Instructions: Blend all the ingredients together until smooth.

12. Spinach Supreme

Ingredients: Spinach, banana, almond butter, coconut milk
Instructions: Blend all the ingredients until creamy and enjoy.

13. Creamy Avocado

Ingredients: Avocado, cucumber, spinach, almond milk
Instructions: Blend the avocado, cucumber, spinach, and almond milk until smooth.

14. Berry Burst

Ingredients: Mixed berries, banana, Greek yogurt, orange juice

Instructions: Blend all the ingredients together until well combined.

15. Mango Madness

Ingredients: Mango, pineapple, coconut milk, honey
Instructions: Blend all the ingredients until creamy and serve.

16. Peanut Butter Power

Ingredients: Banana, peanut butter, spinach, almond milk
Instructions: Blend all the ingredients until smooth and enjoy.

17. Green Energy

Ingredients: Kale, apple, cucumber, lemon, coconut water
Instructions: Blend all the ingredients together until well blended.

18. Chia Delight

Ingredients: Strawberries, chia seeds, almond milk, honey

Instructions: Blend the strawberries, chia seeds, almond milk, and honey until smooth.

19. Peachy Keen

Ingredients: Peaches, Greek yogurt, almond milk, honey

Instructions: Blend all the ingredients together until creamy and serve.

20. Tropical Twist:

Ingredients: Pineapple, banana, coconut water, spinach

Instructions: Blend all the ingredients until well combined and enjoy.

Conclusion

"Anti-Aging Cookbook for Seniors" serves as a culinary compass, guiding individuals towards a healthier and more vibrant aging journey. This remarkable book not only offers a delectable array of nourishing recipes but also empowers seniors to take charge of their well-being. By embracing the power of wholesome ingredients, mindful eating, and age-defying nutrients, seniors can savor the flavors of longevity and vitality.

With each page turned and every meal prepared, this cookbook becomes a trusted ally, reminding us that age is just a number, and our culinary choices can unlock a world of boundless energy and graceful aging.

So, let the kitchen become a sanctuary of rejuvenation, and may the delectable creations within these pages inspire a lifetime of youthful exuberance for all seniors who embark on this flavorful journey.